The Passionate Nurse

by

Liliane de Vries RPN, CPCC

Copyright © 2018 Liliane de Vries
Illustrated by Tomasz "the12" Stasiak

All rights reserved. No part of this publication may be reproduced, distributed, or transmitted in any form or by any means, including photocopying, recording, or other electronic or mechanical methods, without the prior written permission of the publisher, except in the case of brief quotations embodied in critical reviews and certain other non-commercial uses permitted by copyright law. For permission requested, and ordering information please write to the publisher, addressed "Attention: Permissions Coordinator," at the address below.

Alive
103-4001 Bayview Ave
Toronto, Ontario
M2M 327
Canada
www.aliveinhealthcare.com
liliane@aliveinhealthcare.com
Tel: 647-381-7477

Printed in the United States of America
ISBN-13: 978-1978194434
First Edition

I dedicate this book to all the nurses who have put their passion and commitment into caring for others as their priority. I thank them for the long hours and their hard work, especially with the high demands that Nursing requires of them.

Nursing has changed from the times we were able to spend quality time with our patients and connect with them on a human level, to today's evolving demands. With higher expectations, less time, and fewer nurses, we must still find a way to treat our patients as diverse, individual, human beings. Connection, care and humanity are the foundation of the skills we must competently carry out. Nurses are certainly "Champions of Healthcare", and it is my wish, through this book and the work we do at Alive in Healthcare, to remind them that they are just as important as their patients.

Let us all remember to heal ourselves so that we may heal others.

-Liliane de Vries

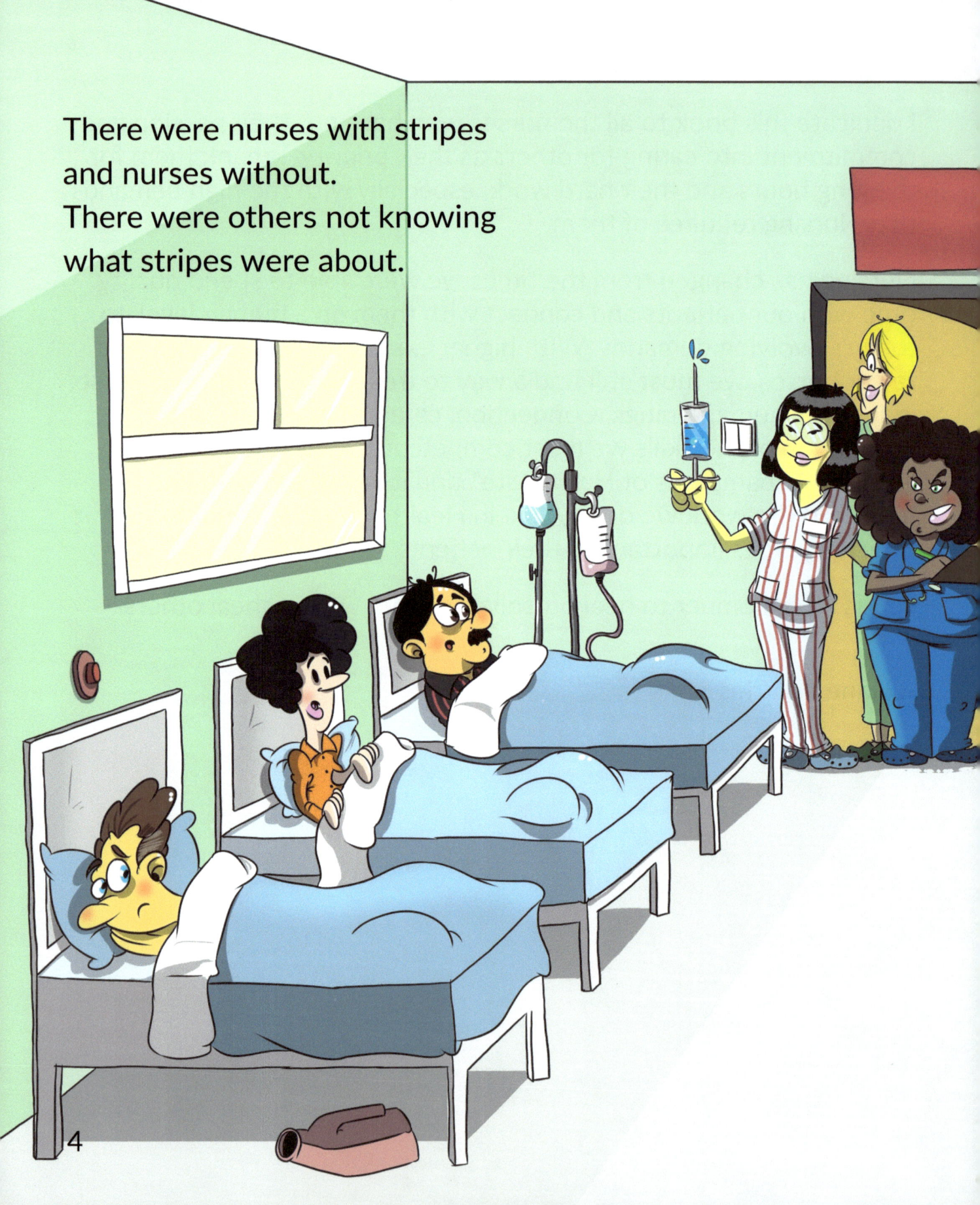

There were nurses with stripes and nurses without.
There were others not knowing what stripes were about.

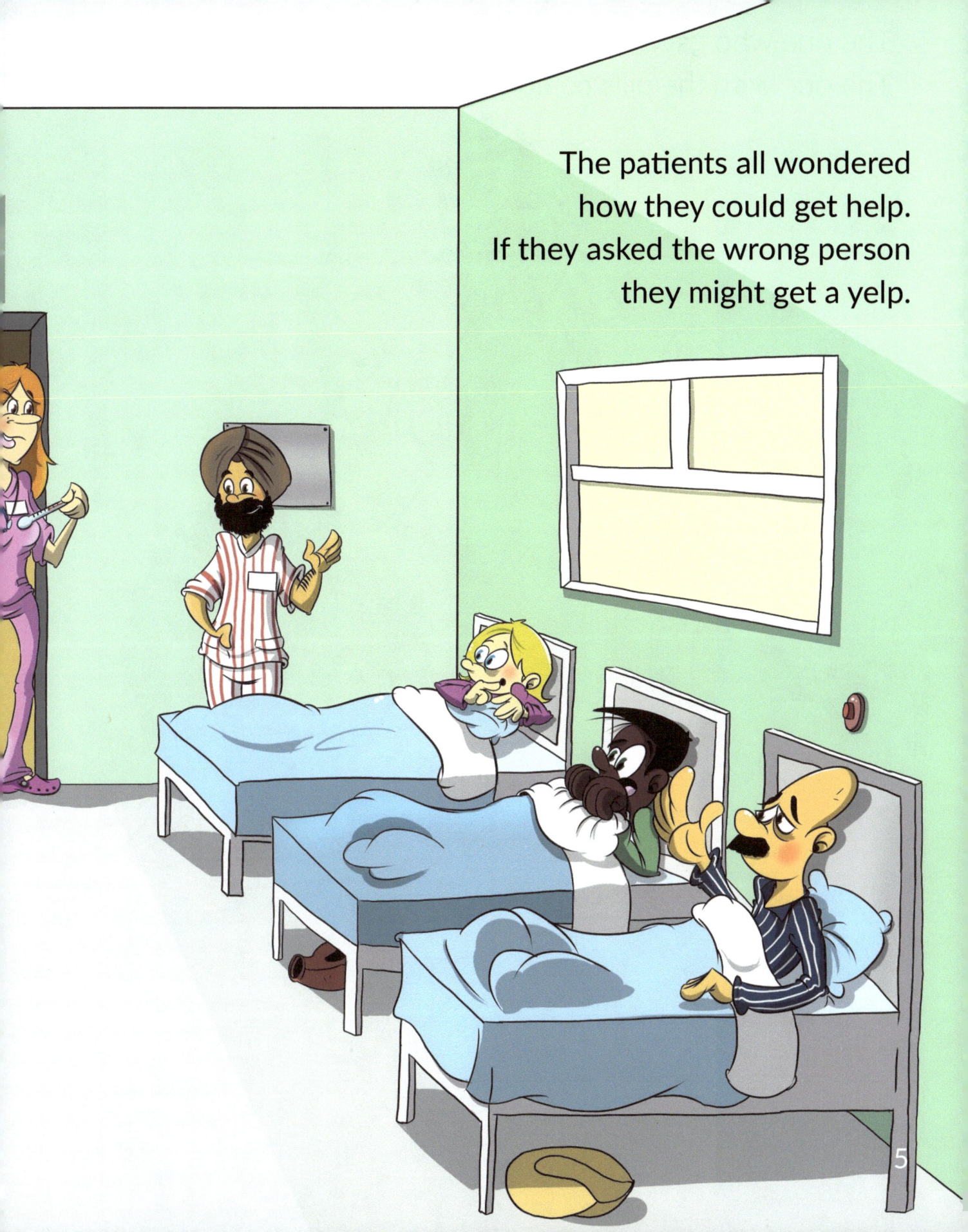

The one who gave bedpans had just cleaned the floor.
The one with the pills could do nothing more.

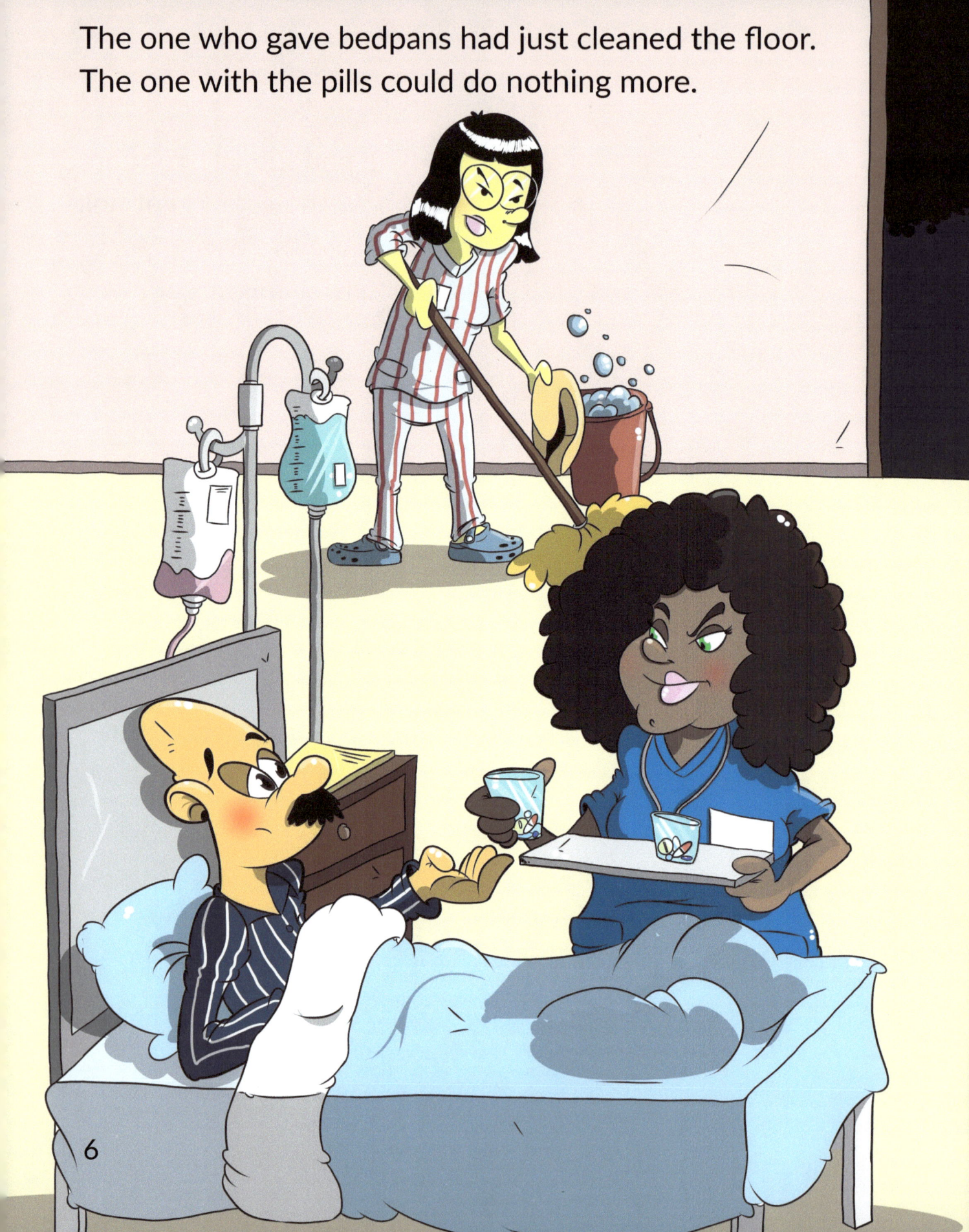

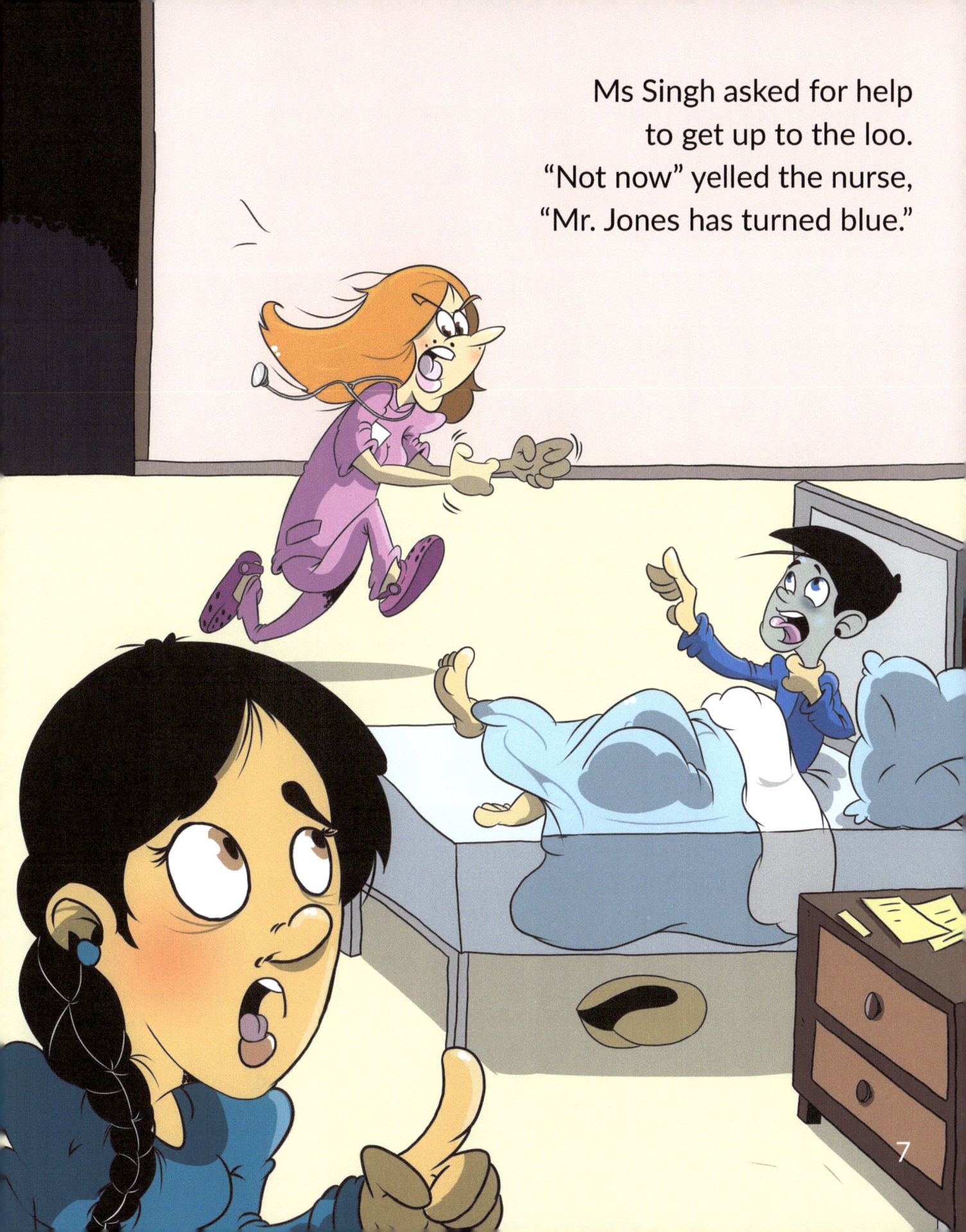

The stripes and the non-stripes complained day and night.
What the others won't do; it looked like a fight.

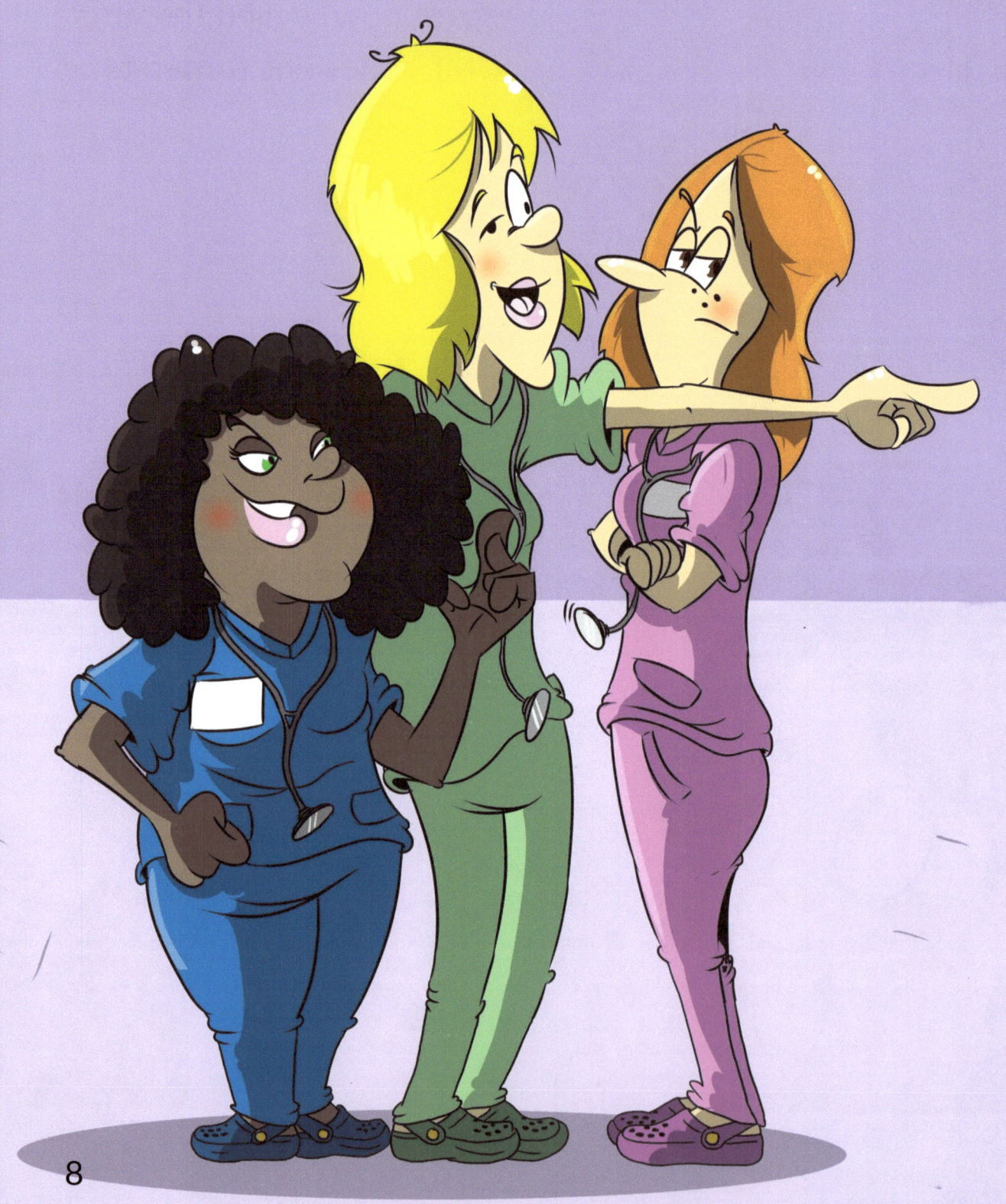

There were no words exchanged to each other at first. But complaining they did; they were making it worse!

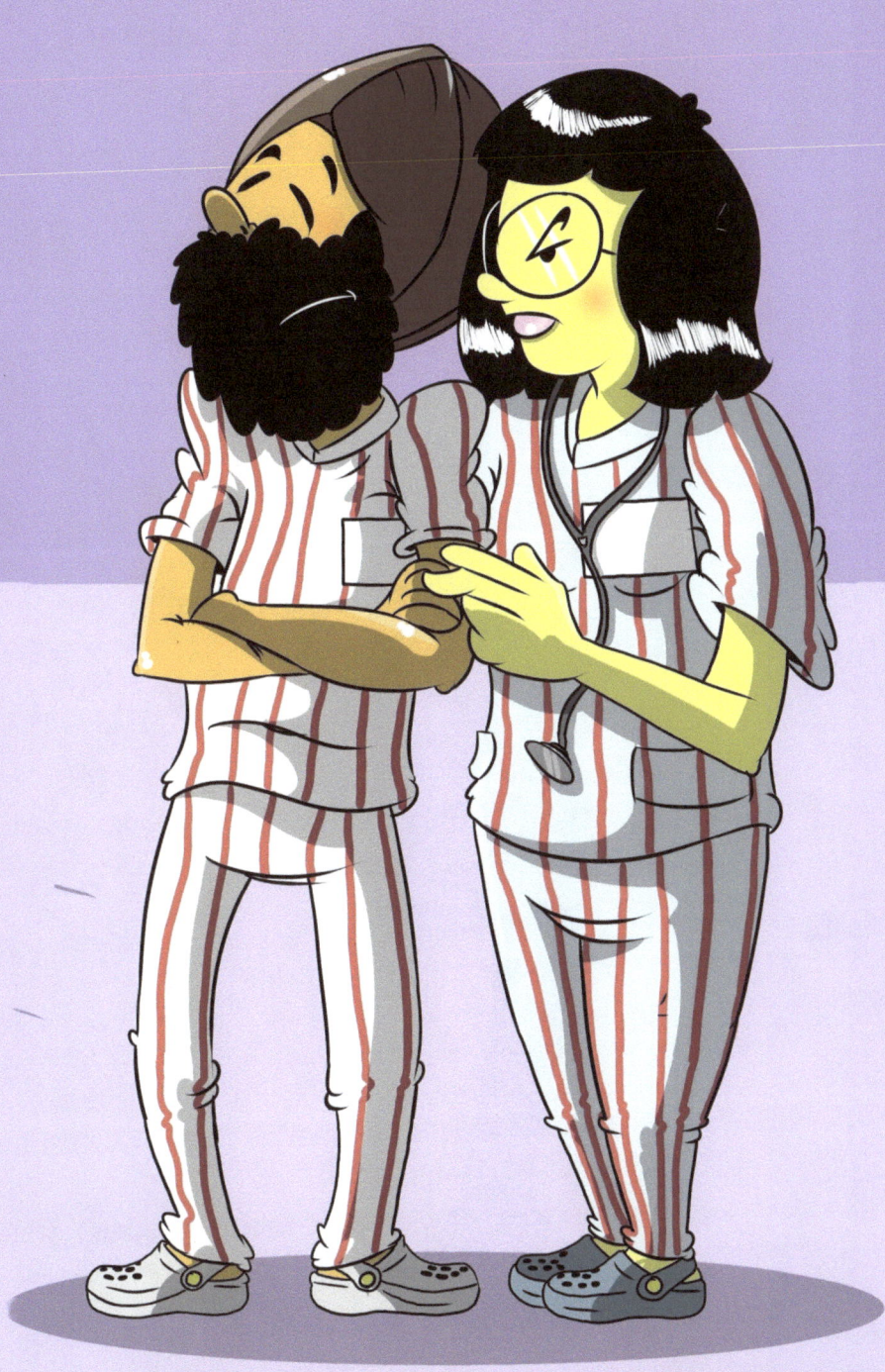

Then one day a stranger came onto the floor,
Different and glowing, with bedpans galore.

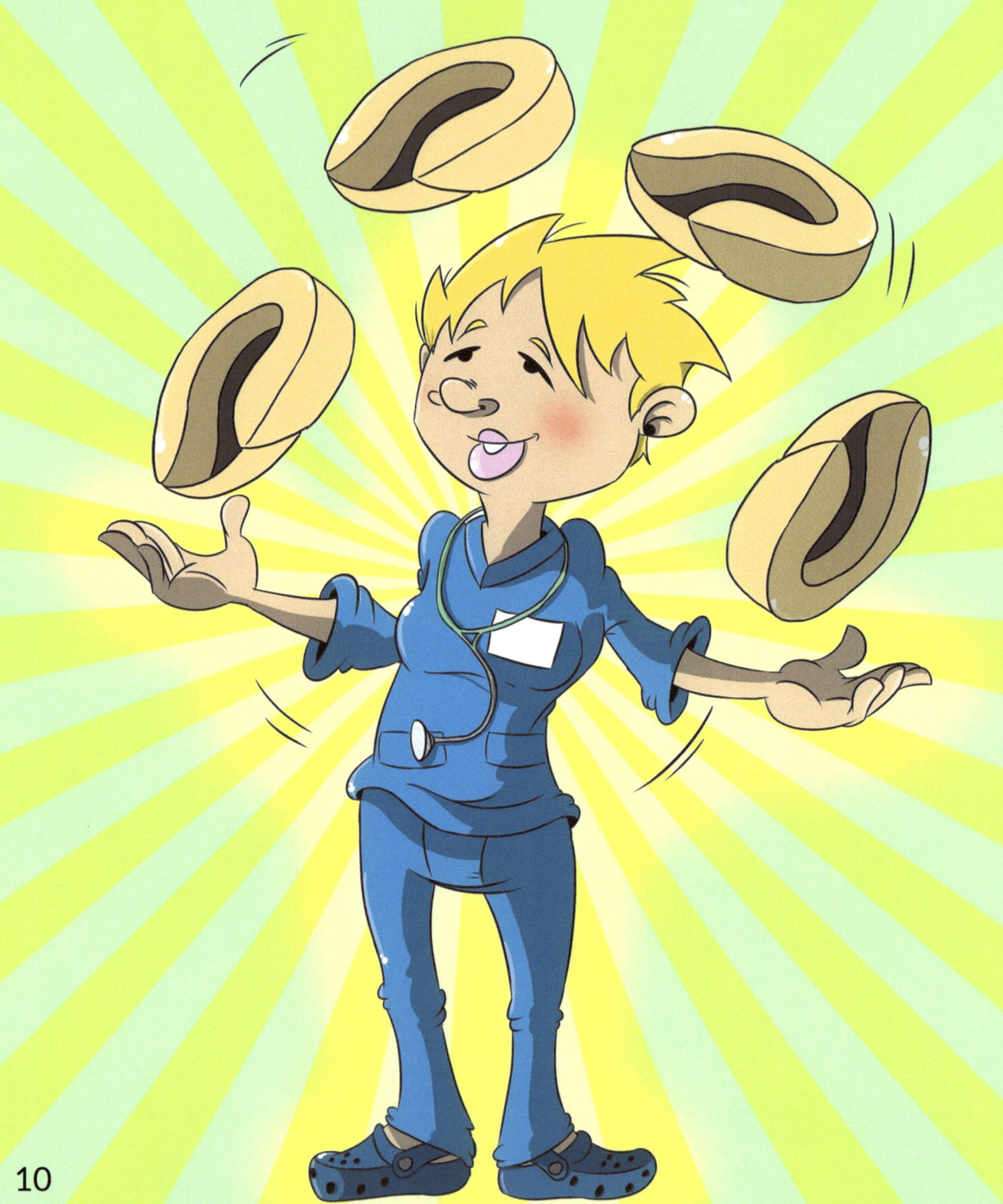

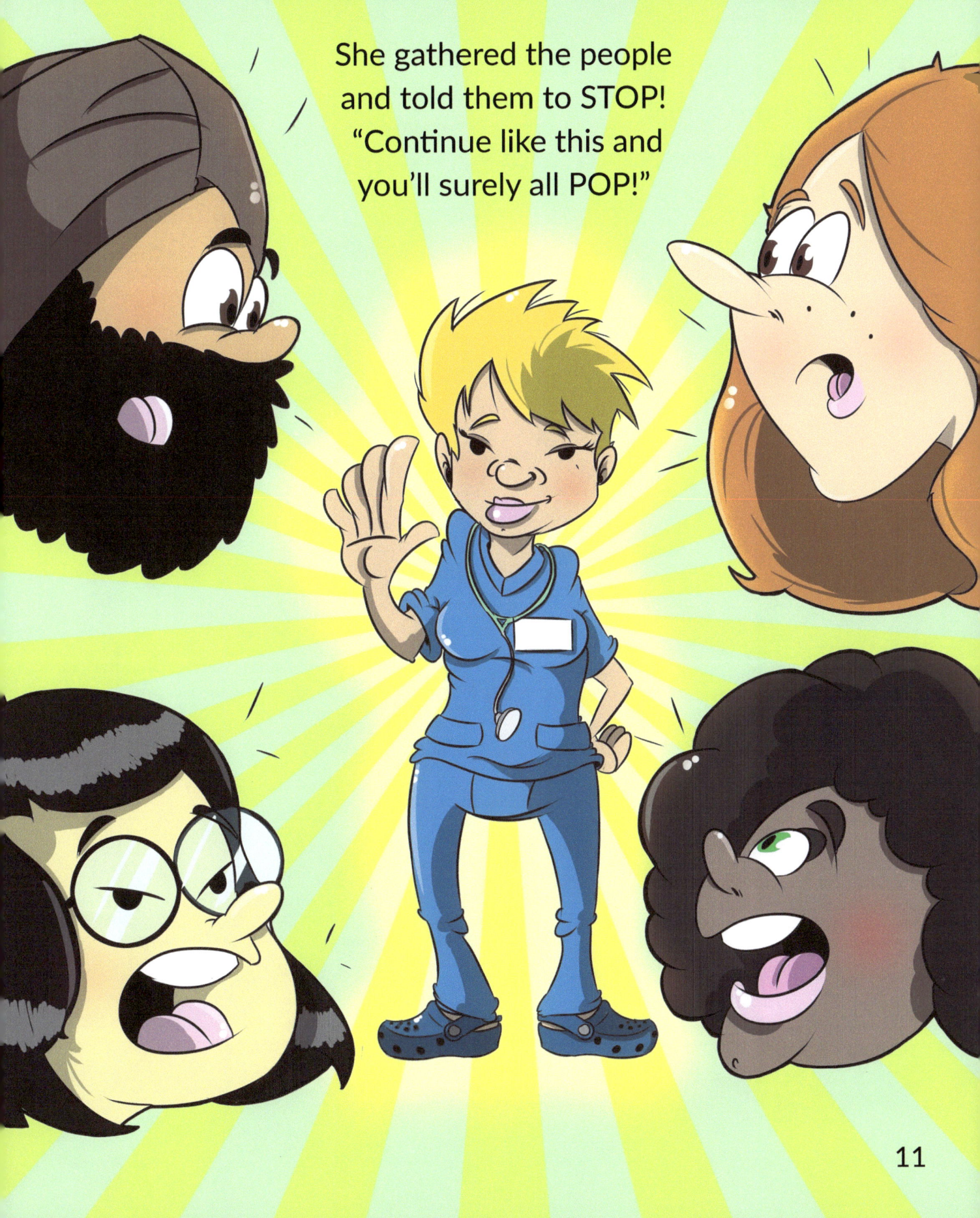

They started to bicker,
complain and attack.
They were different they said;
they were better in fact.

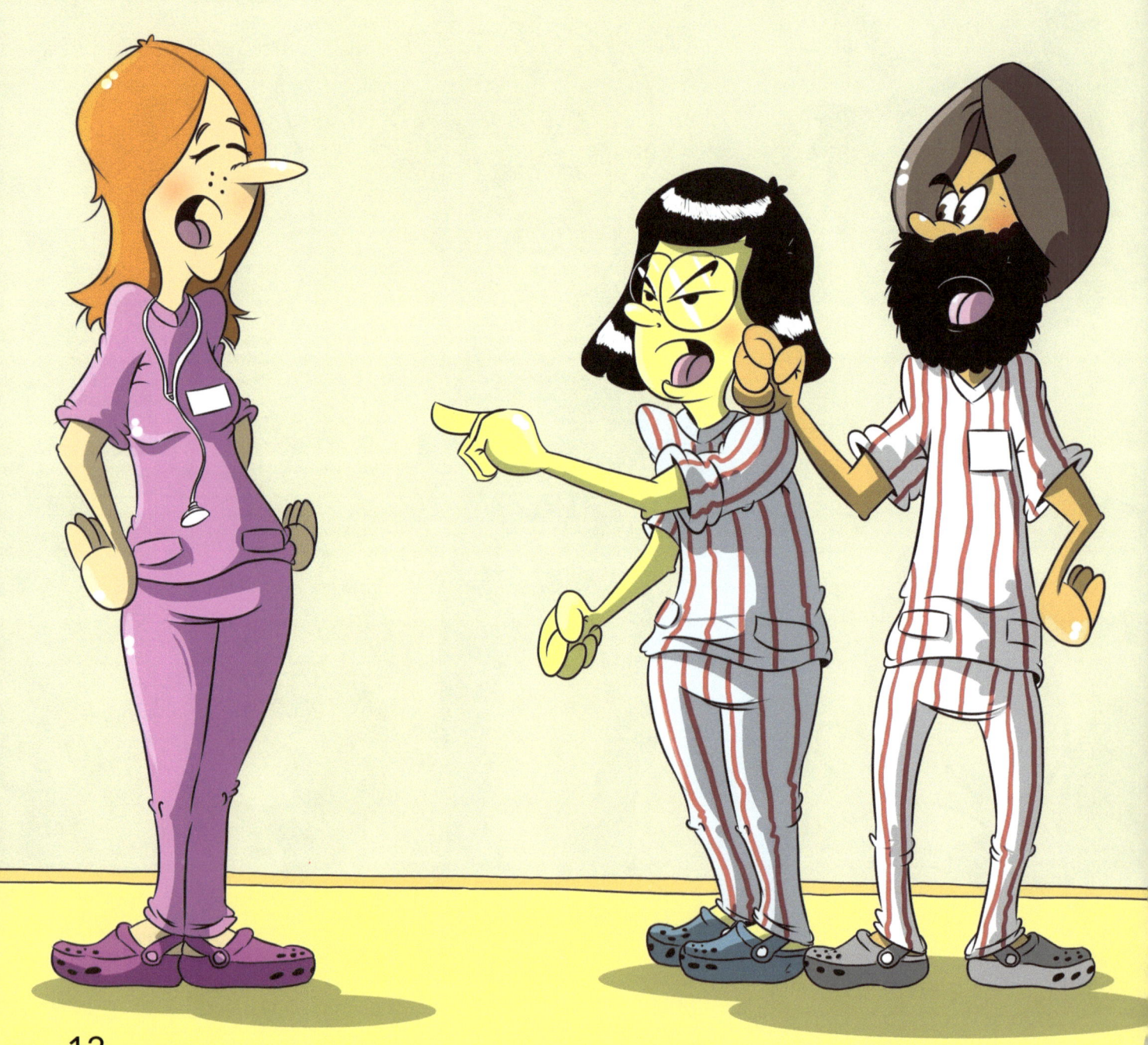

RNs with diplomas; RNs with degrees;
Some older and wiser; some new, here to please.
RPNs with more skills than ever before,
And others who needed to learn so much more.

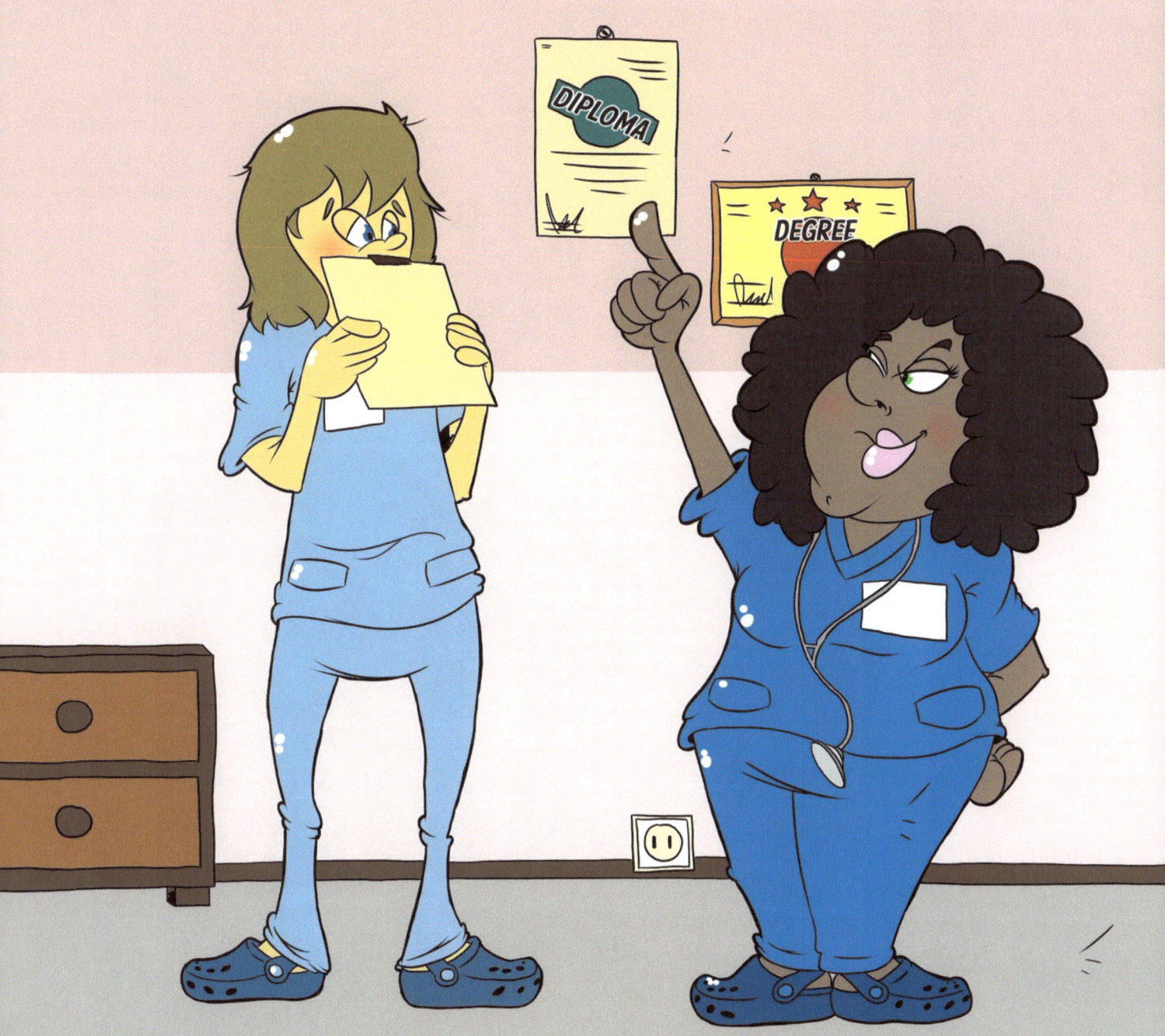

The stranger had come
to ask what they thought.
Did they want to be happy?
Complain 'til they rot'?

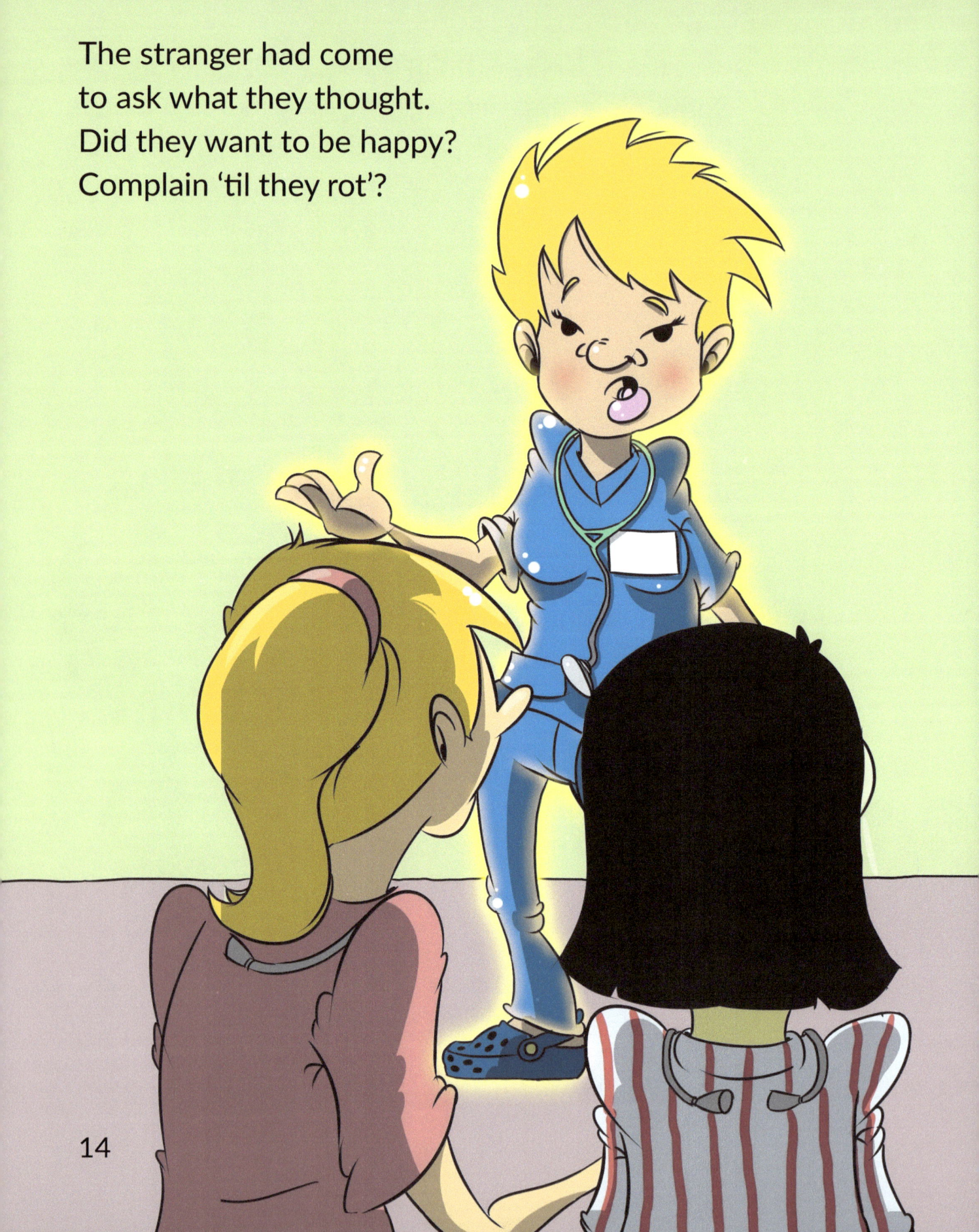

"What brought you to nursing?
What role do you play?
Stripes or no stripes,
you're all humans I say."

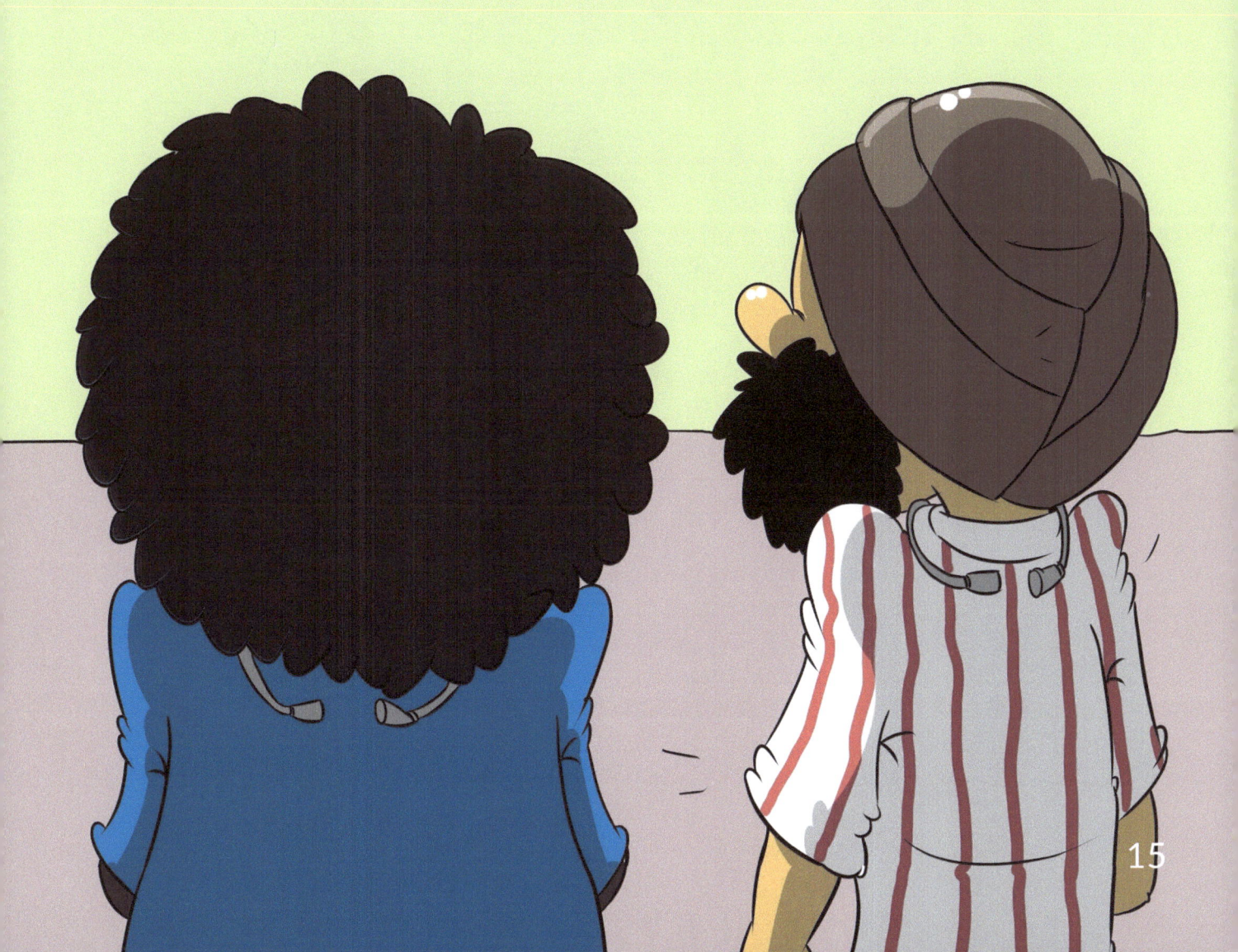

"Don't choose to be victims and blame others too.
Point fingers at healthcare? Too easy to do!

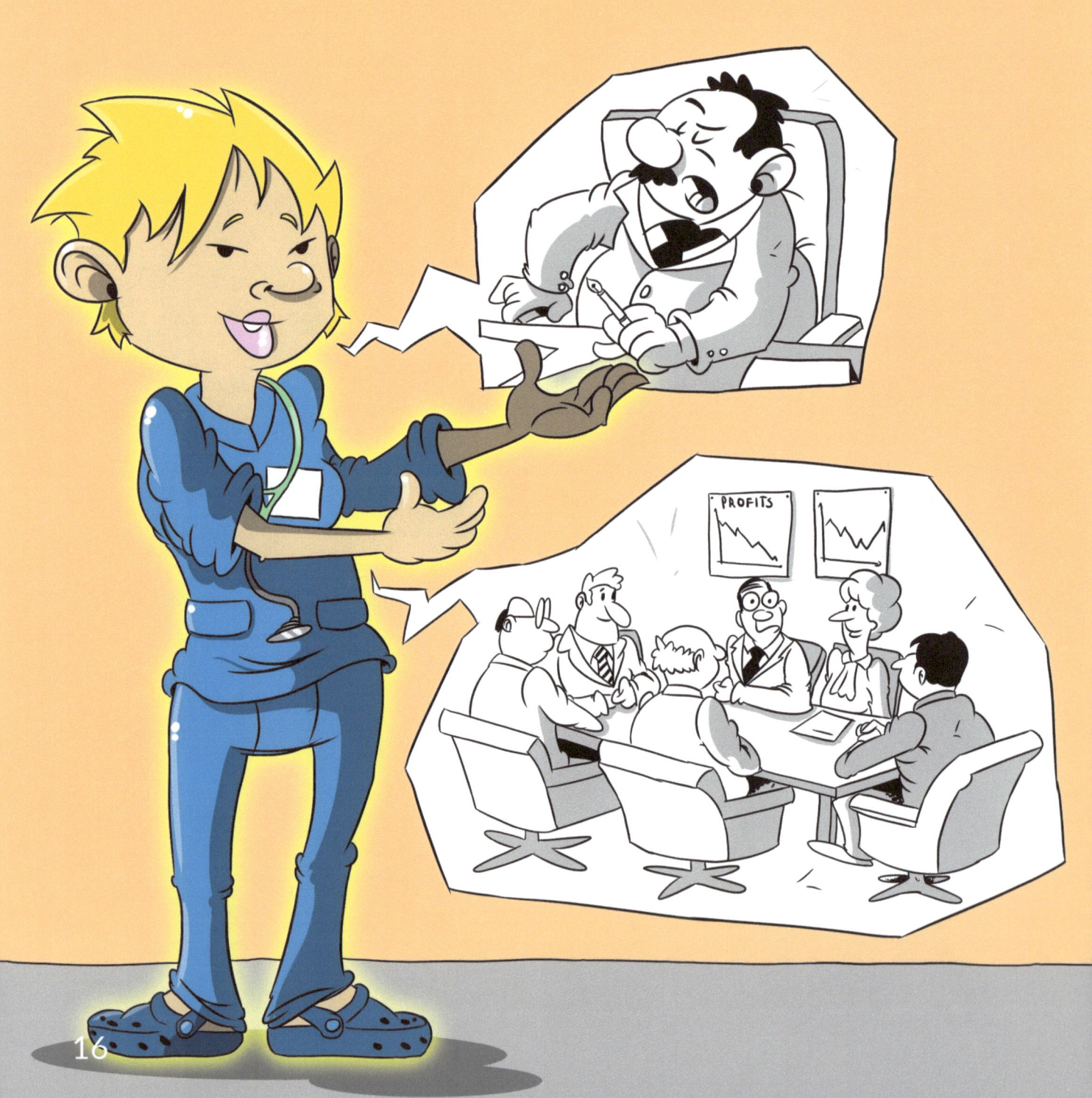

Who suffers the most from the hurt and the pain?
The nurses? The patients? There's nothing to gain!"

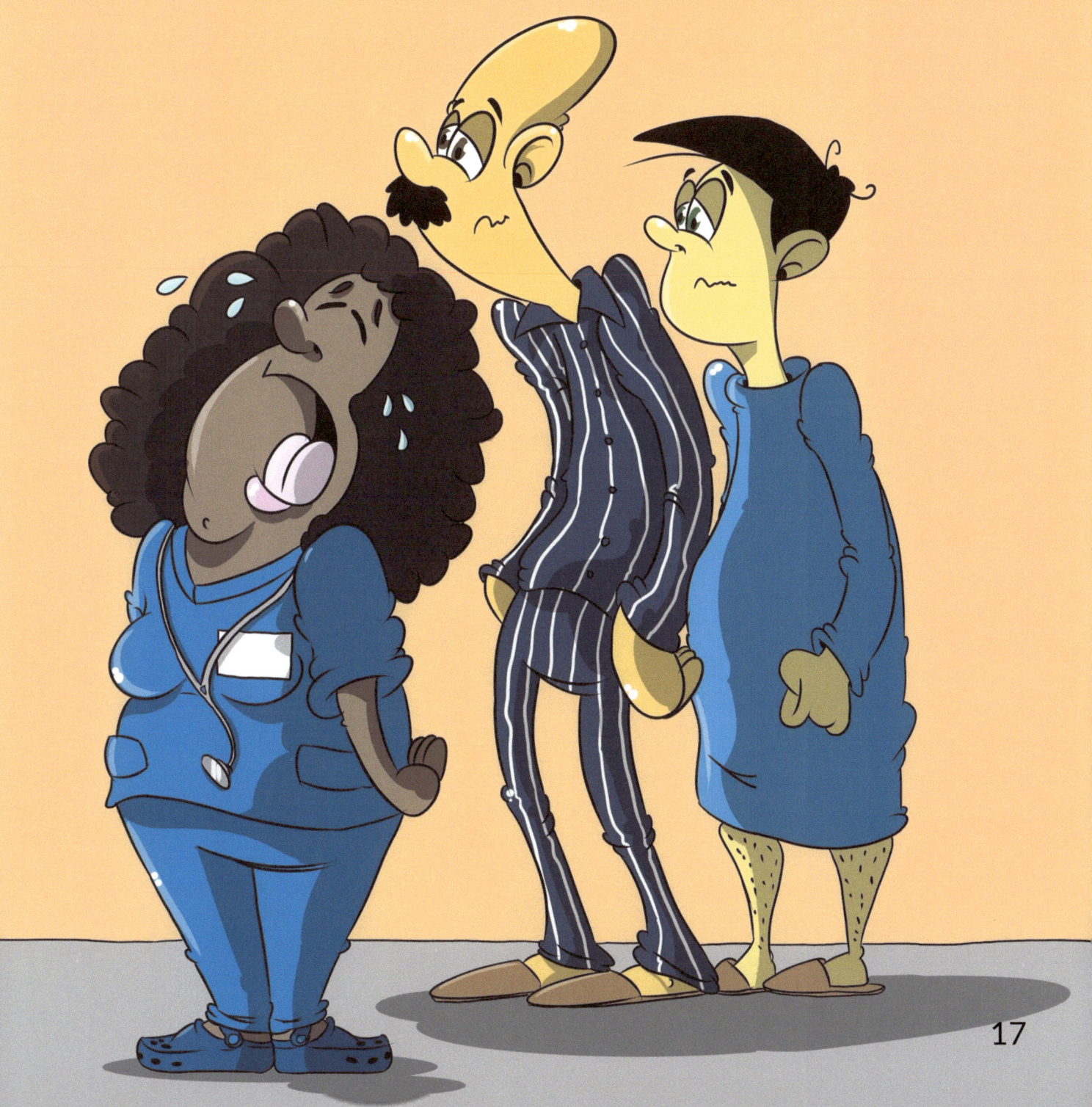

"It's time to take charge" said the stranger that day.
"To change your perspectives; ask questions, I say.

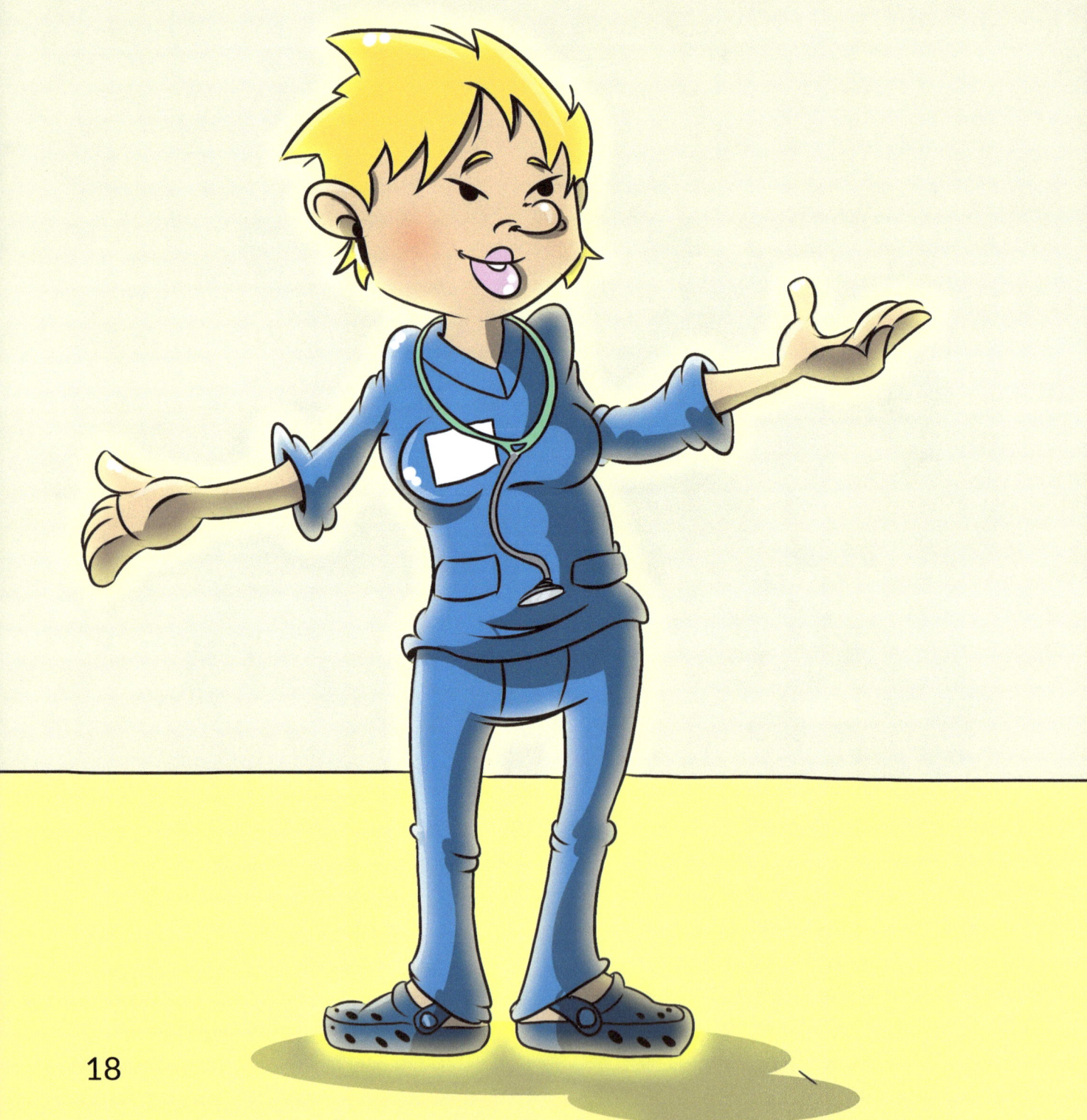

Understand each one's stories,
and listen. Be kind.
The more you can do this,
more time you will find."

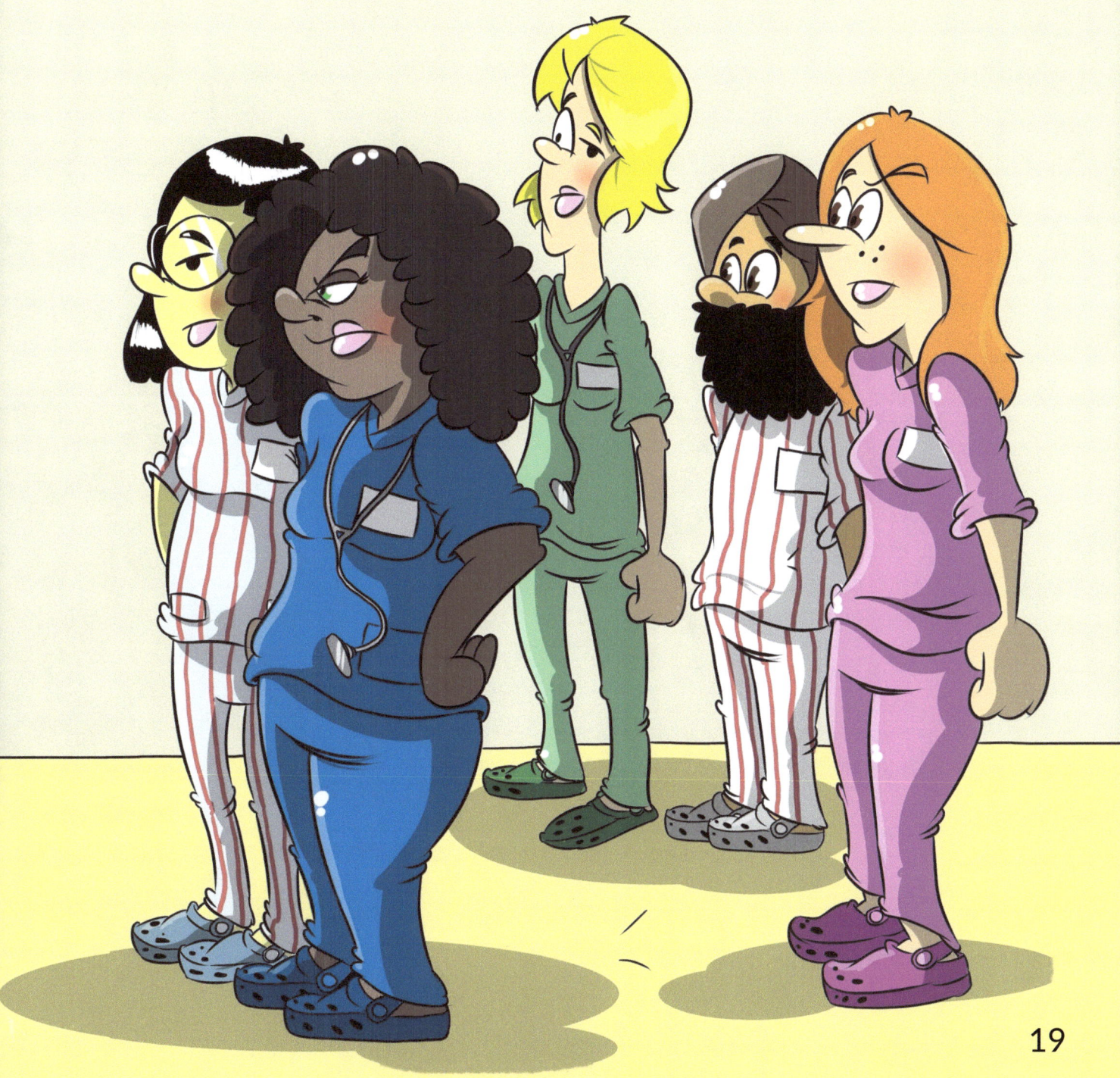

19

"Be helpful, just smile,
and be vulnerable too.
Together we can take
Ms Singh to the loo.

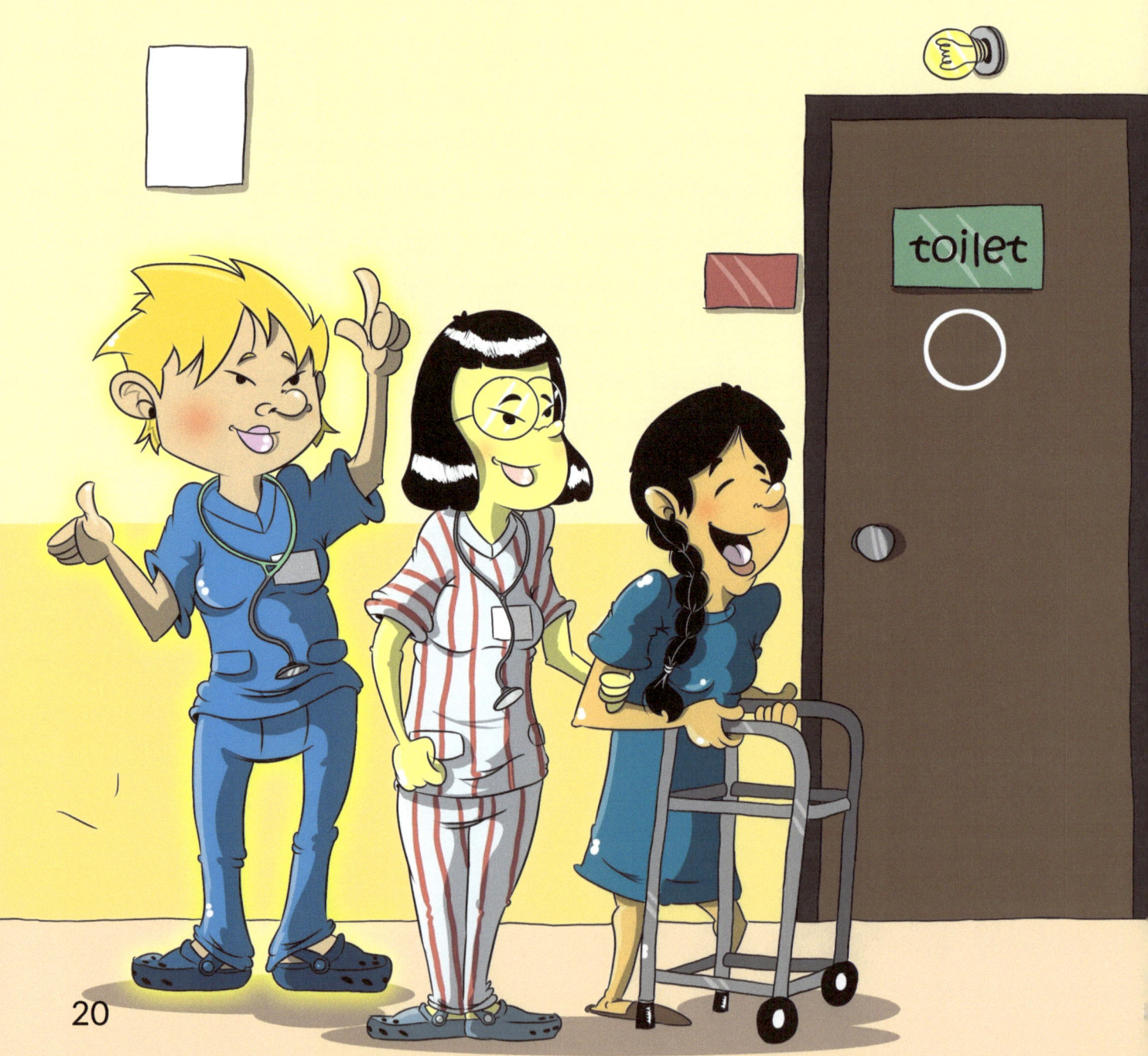

Just say what you need.
Let go; don't be mad.
Reach out to each other;
you'll no longer be sad."

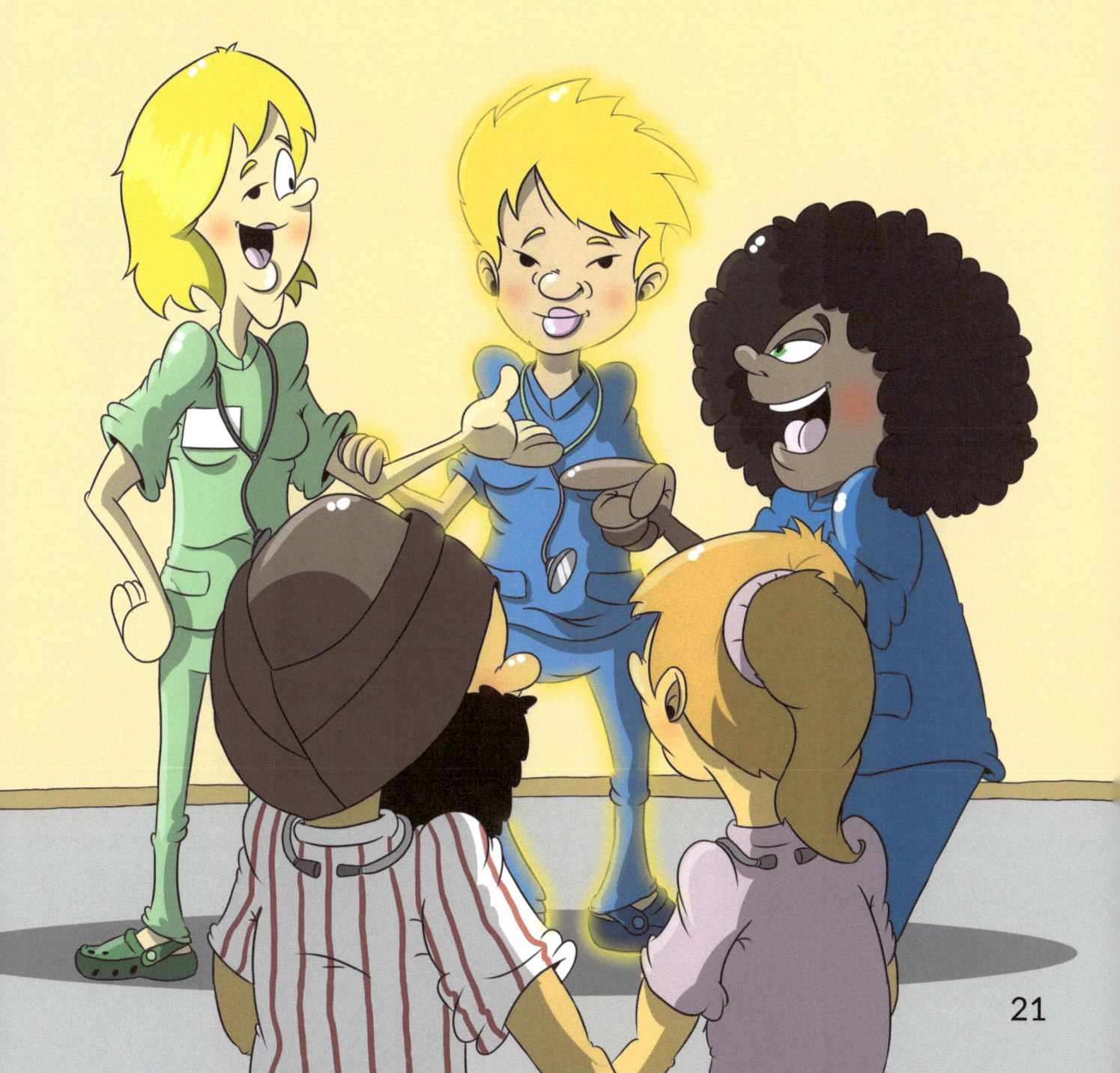

21

"Each one of your voices
deserves to be heard.
You have wisdom, and talent.
Of this I'm assured.

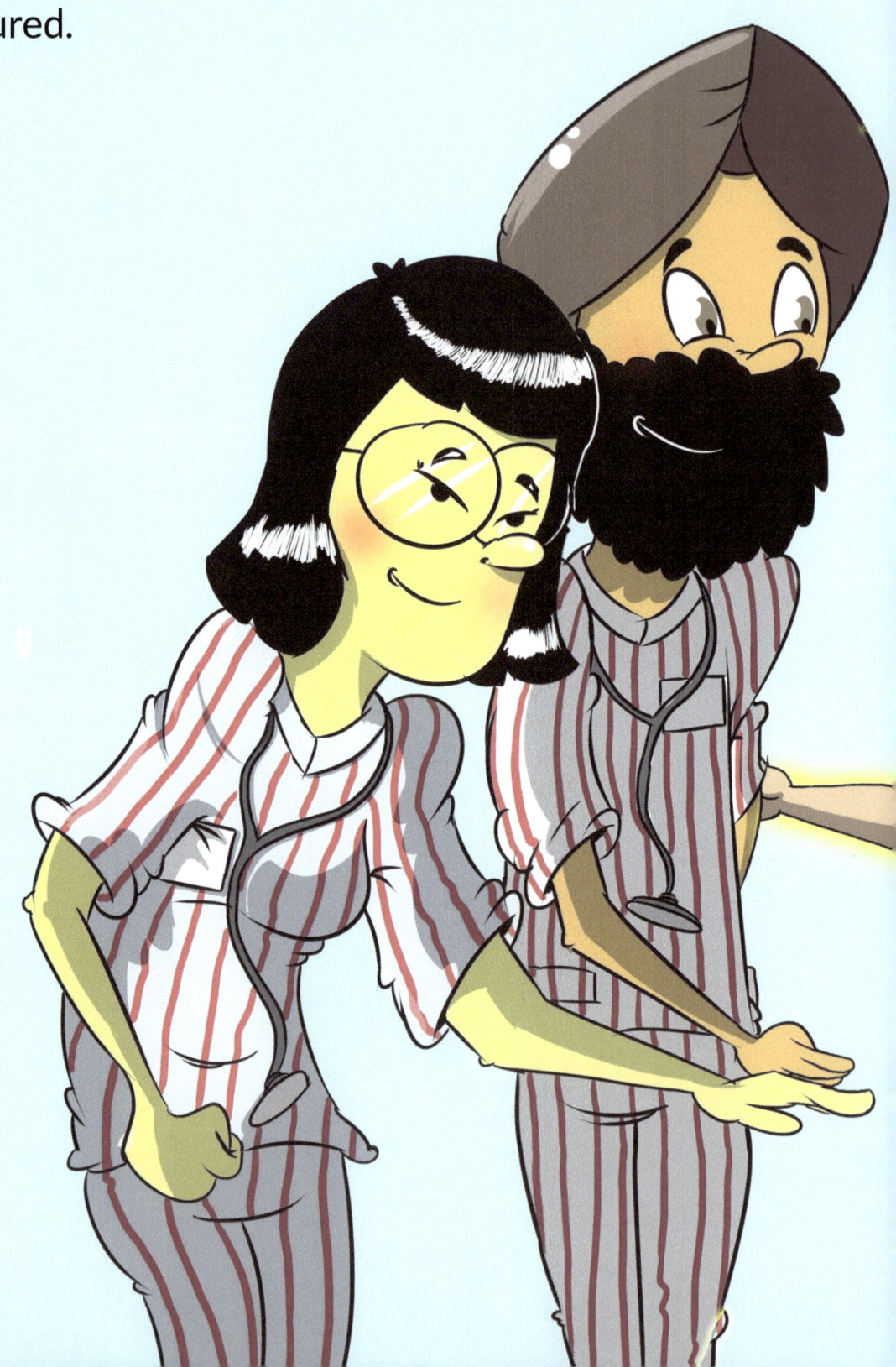

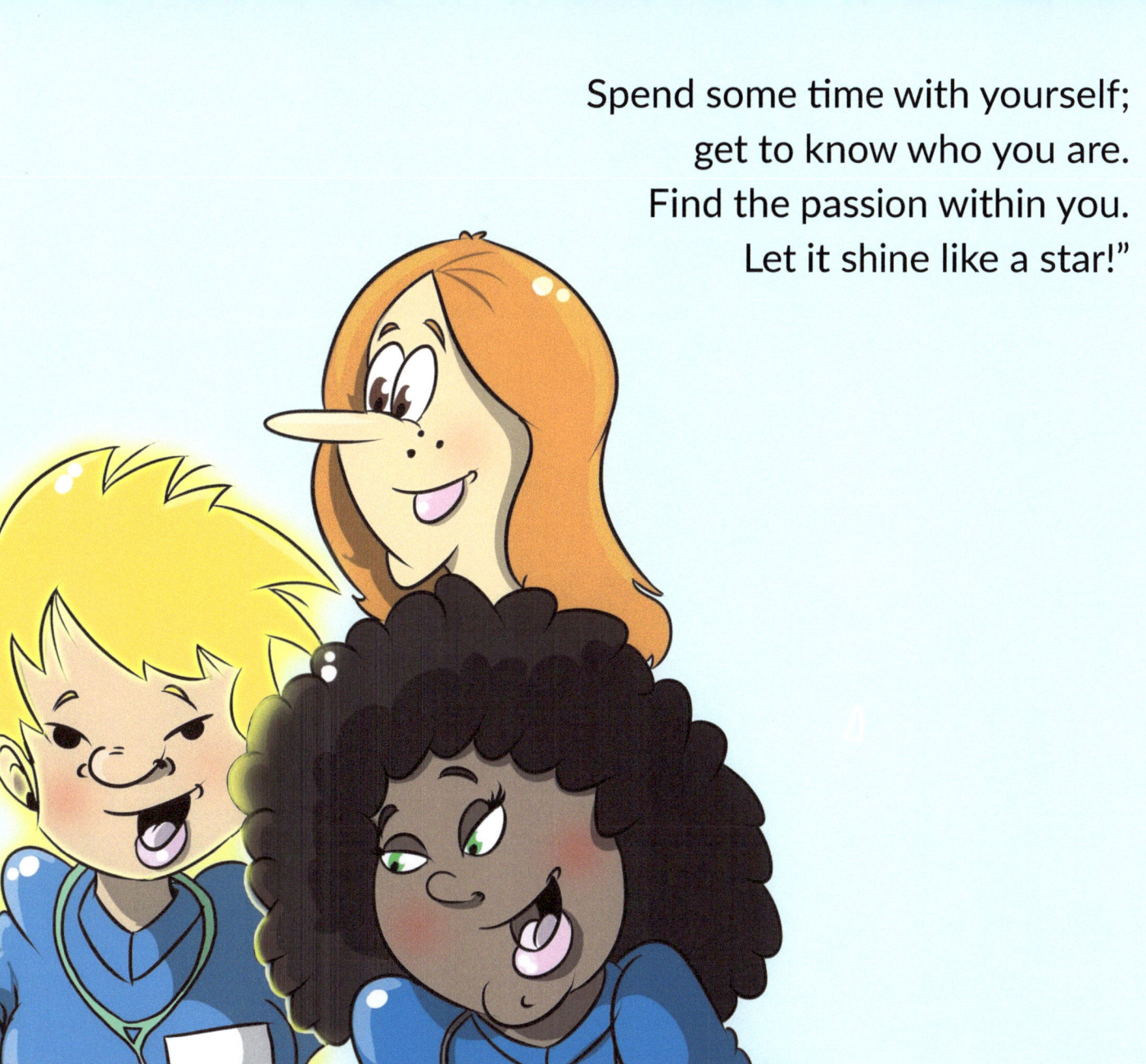

Spend some time with yourself;
get to know who you are.
Find the passion within you.
Let it shine like a star!"

So the stripes they came off, common goals came as one.
They talked and they listened. They even had fun.

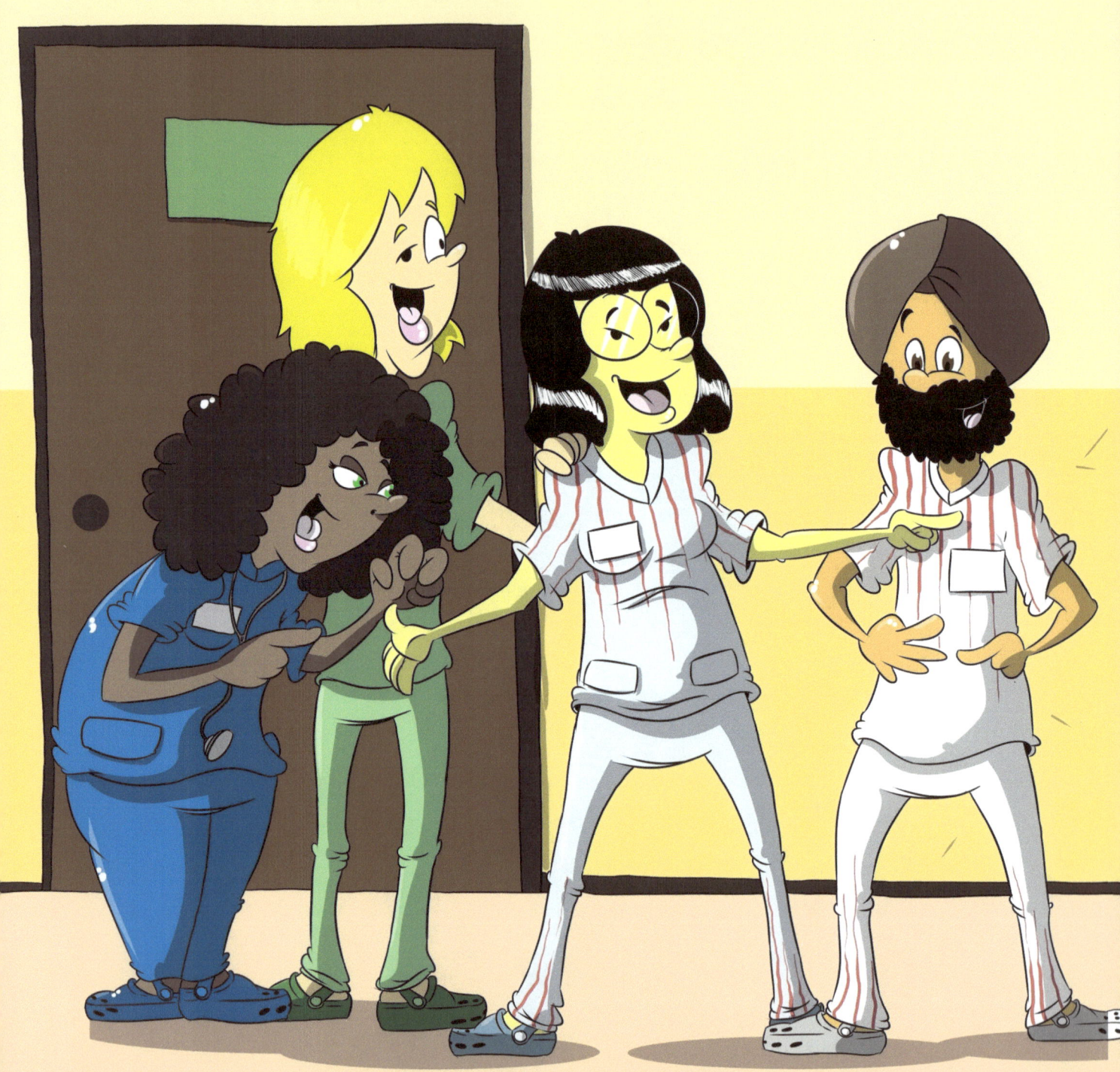

The patients were happy; got the care they deserved. With no righteous opinions, all persons felt heard.

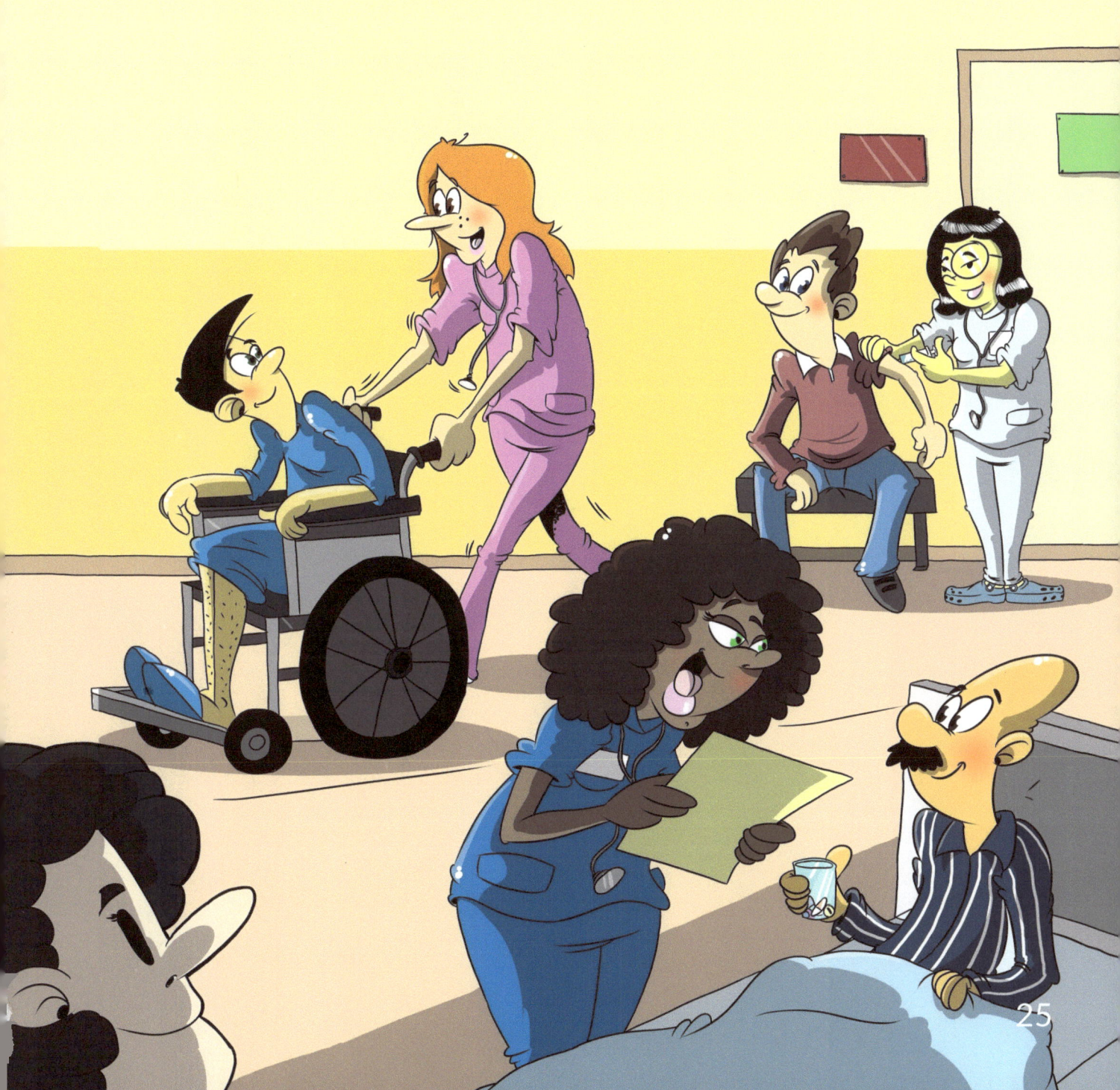

Together they created the culture they wanted.
The stranger had showed them where they had faulted.

All they needed was guidance
to know it was true.

Now the nurses were glowing
and the hospital too.

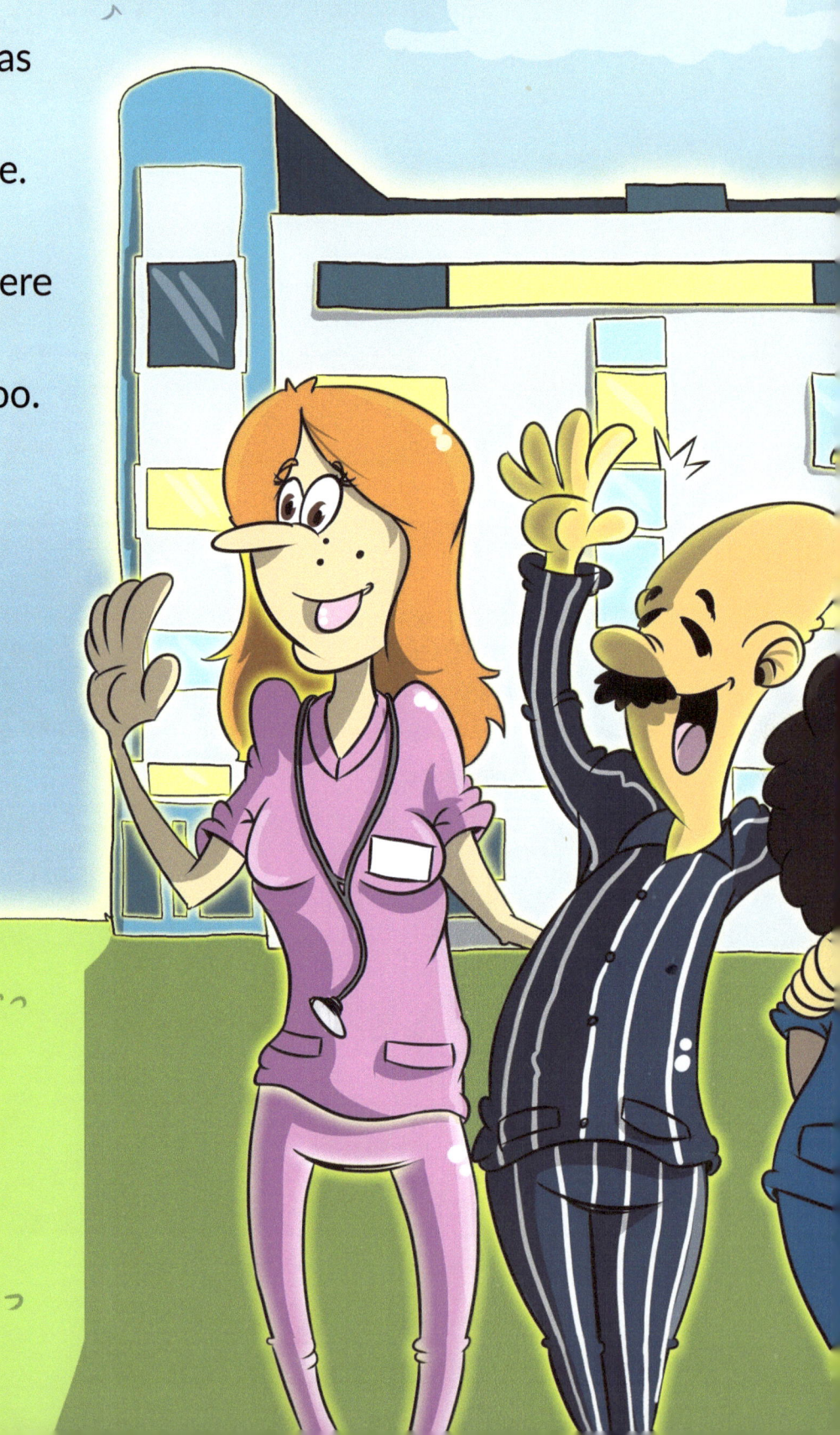

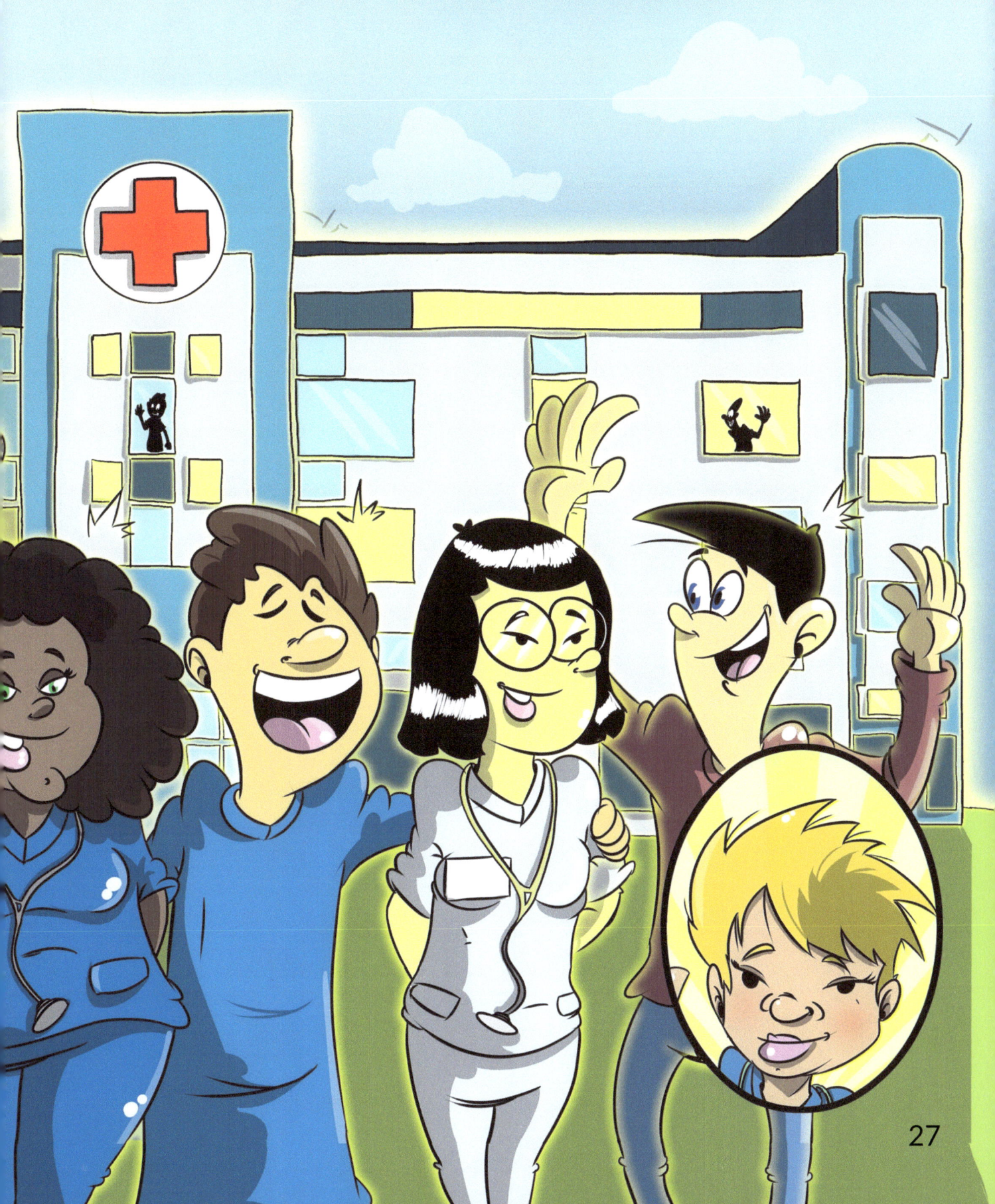